The Diabetic Diary
2004

The Diabetic Diary 2004

L. D. Sutton, M.D., Ph.D.

iUniverse, Inc.

New York Lincoln Shanghai

The Diabetic Diary 2004

iUniverse, Inc.

For information address:
iUniverse
2021 Pine Lake Road, Suite 100
Lincoln, NE 68512
www.iuniverse.com

ISBN: 0-595-29875-3

Printed in the United States of America

Contents

List of Abbreviations

ALT	Alanine aminotransferase
AST	Aspartate aminotransferase
BMI	Body mass index
BUN	Blood urea nitrogen
CK	Creatine Kinase
CRT	Creatinine
dL	deciliter
HDL-C	High density lipoprotein cholesterol
Hg	Mercury
hr	Hour
in	Inches
K	Potassium
Kg	Kilograms
lb	Pounds
LDL-C	Low density lipoprotein cholesterol
m	Meters
meq	Milli-equivalents
mg	Milligrams
min	Minute
mm	Millimeters
Trig	Triglycerides
µg	Micrograms

Introduction

The Centers for Disease control reported in the January 1, 2003 issue of the Journal of the American Medical Association that diabetes increased from 7.3% in 2000 to 7.9% in 2001. That means that over 23 million Americans are afflicted with the disease! That is 1 in 12 of us!

Clearly this is a national epidemic of an unprecedented scale. Secretary of Health and Human Services Tommy G. Thompson has said, "Obesity and diabetes are among our top public health problems in the United States today." And CDC director Dr. Julie L. Gerberding was quoted saying, "These increases are disturbing and are likely even underestimated."

Yet studies continue to show that diabetics are not receiving adequate care and education. Scientific clinical studies continue and have provided the foundations for a well-defined, but rather complex regimen for health maintenance management of diabetics. *The Diabetic Diary 2003* simplifies this regimen and is the means by which the diabetic patient can take control of his/her own medical management.

Myths about diabetes abound. I frequently meet diabetic patients who tell me they have to avoid carbohydrates and sugar. This is patently wrong! A diet wherein less than 50 to 60% of calories are derived from carbohydrates is a diet that enhances diabetic complications and mortality. And sugar should be counted just the same as any other carbohydrate! See the dietary section on page 19.

Very frequently I meet type 2 diabetic patients who do not check their blood sugars often, if at all. If these patients aren't measuring their home blood sugars and recording them, then how then can they or their doctors know if their prescribed medications are working properly?

There is not a lot of reading in this book, but what is here is important. The text concisely and simply summarizes general treatment goals for the diabetic patient. Read the text and review it often. Knowing the information in this book will keep you well ahead of the pack with respect to diabetic management.

Most importantly, fill out the tables in this book. Diabetic management requires diligence. Check your blood sugars often and record them. Get your laboratory testing done on schedule and record the results. Get your examinations done and record them. If you do this, you and your doctor will be able to readily determine if you're meeting your health maintenance goals.

This book is not intended to prescribe treatment. Because treatment must be individualized, you should consult with your physician for recommendations concerning your treatment requirements. But this book will go far in ensuring you get the proper medical maintenance management.

Thank you for choosing *THE DIABETIC DIARY 2003*. It is an honor to be chosen to participate in your health care delivery.

PERSONAL INFORMATION

▶ Fill in the information as directed.

▶ **Take this book with you for all physician and emergency room visits.** The information in this section, and the Past Medical History and Medications sections provide important and sometimes critical information to health care providers concerning your medical management. The information as presented in this book is designed to be as efficient as possible for your physicians.

▶ Diabetes that was formerly referred to as Juvenile, Type I or Insulin Dependent is now correctly referred to as **Type 1**.

▶ Diabetes that was formerly referred to as Adult, Type II or Non-insulin Dependent is now correctly referred to as **Type 2**.

▶ There are other types under special medical circumstances. If your disease is not Type 1 or Type 2, then fill in your specific diagnosis.

Name
Date of birth _____
Date first diagnosed with diabetes _____
Type 1 or 2 diabetes? (circle one) or List other type: _____
List **allergies** to medicines: _____
_____
_____
_____

Do you use **insulin** to control your diabetes? YES or NO
Current address: _____
_____
_____
_____

EMERGENCY NOTIFICATION:
Name _____
Address _____
_____
_____

Telephone number _____
PERSONAL PHYSICIAN: Name _____
Telephone number _____

MEDICAL AND SURGICAL HISTORY

▶ Fill in the information as directed. Just check mark the diseases that you have or have had. Leave the rest of the spaces blank. This will allow you to check mark additional diagnosis as they occur.

▶ While this section is designed to give your doctor the past medical history pertinent to your health care, space is left at the end of this section for additional history. You may also use this section to elaborate on the diagnosis you check. For example you may list the number and dates of each heart attack or your bypass operation or your stroke(s).

▶ Please keep this section as legible as possible. Clutter may lead to misinterpretation and compromise your medical outcome.

Medical History

Tobacco: Currently smoke _____ packs of cigarettes per day.

Quit smoking in the year _____

I use other tobacco products. _____

I have never used tobacco products _____

I have _____ **alcoholic** drinks per DAY / WEEK / OCCASIONAL.

Check all diagnosis that apply:

Stroke (Brain attack) _____

Transient ischemic attacks (TIA, mini-strokes) _____

Stroke (Cerebral Hemorrhage) _____

Seizures (epilepsy) _____

Coronary artery disease(Heart disease) _____

Previous heart attacks _____

Angina _____

Congestive heart failure _____

Heart valve disease _____

Mitral valve prolapse _____

High blood pressure _____

Arrhythmia (irregular heart beat) _____

Peripheral vascular disease (claudication) _____

Deep venous thrombosis (DVT) _____

Cataracts _____

Diabetic retinopathy _____

Macular degeneration _____

Legally blind _____

Asthma _____

COPD (Emphysema) _____

Diabetic gastroparesis _____

Heart burn (GERD) _____

Hiatal hernia _____

Peptic ulcer disease _____

Gastrointestinal (GI) bleeding _____

Diverticulitis _____

Irritable bowel syndrome _____

Hernia _____

Kidney disease _____

Diabetic foot disease _____

Number of pregnancies _____

Number of deliveries _____
Number of miscarriages _____
Diabetic neuropathy _____
Obesity _____
Osteoarthritis _____
Rheumatoid arthritis _____
Lupus erythmatosis _____
Osteoporosis _____
Hypothyroidism _____
Hyperparathyroidism _____
Addison's disease _____
Liver failure _____
Gall stones (cholelithiasis) _____
Gall bladder inflammation (cholecystitis) _____
Compression fractures _____
Cancers:
    Brain tumor _____
    Breast _____
    Lung _____
    Colon _____
    Prostate _____
    Cervical _____
    Uterine _____
    Ovarian _____
    Testicular _____
    Kidney _____
    Bladder _____
    Liver _____
    Pancreas _____
    Thyroid _____
    Multiple endocrine neoplasia _____
    Leukemia _____
    Lymphoma _____
    Skin, melanoma _____
    Skin, basal cell _____
    Skin, squamous cell _____
Infectious disease:
    HIV positive _____
    AIDS _____
    Hepatitis A _____

Hepatitis B   ———
Hepatitis C   ———
Hepatitis, non-A, non-B, non-C   ———
Rheumatic fever   ———
Additions, clarifications and hospitalizations:

_____

_____

_____

_____

_____

_____

_____

_____

_____

_____

_____

_____

_____

SURGICAL HISTORY

Check all procedures that apply:

Appendectomy _____

Gall bladder (cholecystectomy) _____

Cataract repair _____

Colonoscopy _____

Upper endoscopy (EGD) _____

Tonsillectomy _____

Adenoidectomy _____

Cesarean section _____

Coronary artery bypass graft (CABG, Heart bypass) _____

Cardiac catheterization (angiography) _____

Coronary artery angioplasty (balloon) _____

Coronary artery stent placement _____

Bone marrow biopsy _____

Breast biopsy _____

Breast lumpectomy _____

Mastectomy _____

Transurethral retrograde prostatectomy (TURP) _____

Prostatectomy _____

Bone marrow biopsy _____

Liver transplant _____

Heart transplant _____

Kidney transplant _____

Pancreas transplant _____

Bone marrow transplant _____

Bone transplant (autologous) _____

Skin graft _____

Sinus surgery _____

Lung tumor removal _____

Lung lobectomy _____

Brain tumor removed _____

Femoral-popliteal bypass graft _____

Splenectomy _____

Dental extraction _____

List other operations and surgical procedures:

_____

_____

CURRENT MEDICATIONS

▶ List the names of your medications, dosage and times of day taken. If you take different doses of the same medication at different times, feel free to list these on separate lines. Again, legibility counts.

▶ In the insulin section fill in only those that apply and leave the rest blank. For specialized regimens, sliding scale regimens and insulin pump settings be as exact and legible as possible; giving type of insulin and when administered.

▶ Generally a diabetic should be on medications to control blood sugar, a daily aspirin, lipid controlling medications and possibly blood pressure medications with special preference towards medications called angiotensin converting enzyme (ACE) inhibitors for renal (kidney) protection. Check with your physician.

CURRENT MEDICATIONS

Name of Medicine	Dosage	Taken Times Daily
_____	_____	_____
_____	_____	_____
_____	_____	_____
_____	_____	_____
_____	_____	_____
_____	_____	_____
_____	_____	_____
_____	_____	_____
_____	_____	_____
_____	_____	_____
_____	_____	_____
_____	_____	_____
_____	_____	_____

Name of **INSULIN** used: _____

Regular	Morning units _____	Evening units _____
NPH (Lente)	Morning units _____	Evening units _____
Ultra Lente	Morning units _____	Evening units _____
70/30	Morning units _____	Evening units _____
Humulin	Morning units: _____	Evening units _____

Insulin pump settings: _____

_____

_____

Sliding scale and specialized regimens: _____

_____

_____

_____

_____

_____

_____

_____

_____

_____

_____

_____

_____

_____

_____

_____

IMMUNIZATIONS

▸ Enter the dates for your most recent vaccination(s).

▸ Diabetics are considered to have impaired immune function. Therefore, they may have worse cases of infectious diseases, making them sicker and increasing likelihood of death. Immunizations play an important role in diabetic management.

▸ At a minimum diabetics should have:
  1) An annual influenza vaccination.
  2) One lifetime pneumococcus vaccination.
  3) Current tetanus vaccination.

Influenza

▸ Vaccinate annually. Each year 20 million Americans catch the flu and **44,000** of them die! Were you worried about SARS?

▸ All diabetic patients should receive an annual influenza vaccine beginning each September. Contra-indications include allergy to egg products or other components of the influenza vaccine and Guillain-Barré syndrome within 6 weeks of a previous influenza vaccination. The vaccination cannot cause influenza or other respiratory diseases. The most common side effect is soreness at the injection site.

▸ Prophylaxis with anti-influenza drugs such as Symmetrel (amantadine) and Flumadine (rimantadine) may be used if allergy prevents immunization. These drugs are effective only against Influenza A. Tamiflu (oseltamivir) is approved for prophylaxic use. To date Relenza (zanamivir) is only approved for treatment of influenza infections, but presumably would be effective as an influenza prophylactic. Tamiflu and Relenza are effective against both Influenza A & B.

▸ *Influenza vaccination does not guarantee that one will not catch the flu!*
   1. The trivalent vaccine is constituted of strains of Influenza A & B most likely to circulate in the USA during influenza season. Exposure to another strain of influenza might result in infection.
   2. A vaccinated patient may become infected with a strain immunized against, but the disease should not be as severe.
   3. Many other viruses cause influenza-like symptoms, but are generally referred to as "the flu."

Influenza vaccination date _____/_____/_____

Pneumococcus

▸ A.K.A. Streptococcus pneumoniae. One time vaccination.

▸ All diabetics should receive at least one pneumococcal vaccination. Indications for repeat vaccination include:
  1. Patients over the age of 65 that were less than 65 years old at the time of their initial vaccination *and* more than 5 years have elapsed since their initial vaccination.
  2. Other indications for repeat vaccination may include nephrotic syndrome, chronic renal disease and immunocompromised states.

▸ Up to half of patients receiving pneumococcal vaccination experience soreness at the injection site. Severe reactions are rare.

▸ It is well established that the pneumococcal vaccine is effective in reducing life threatening disease due to pneumococcal blood infection (pneumococcal bacteremia). Its effectiveness in preventing other pneumococcal disease remains uncertain, including pneumococcal pneumonia. One should also remember that other bacteria and viruses can cause pneumonia. *It is therefore a misnomer to refer to this vaccination as the "pneumonia shot!"*

Pneumococcal vaccination date(s):#1_____/_____/_____
#2 _____/_____/_____

Tetanus

▸ Boost every 10 years. Complete series may be indicated.

▸ Diphtheria-tetanus toxoid should be administered every 10 years. If over 30 years have elapsed or if one has never been immunized, the whole series should be administered. Contra-indications to tetanus vaccination include allergy to any component of the vaccine.

Tetanus vaccination date:
#1 _____/_____/_____
#2 _____/_____/_____
#3 _____/_____/_____

DIETARY RECOMMENDA-TIONS
Medical Nutrition Therapy

▸ Dietary recommendations have changed dramatically during the past century resulting in much confusion amongst physicians. The following is what the American Diabetic Association currently recommends.

▸ **Calorie Reduction:** A modest calorie reduction of 250 to 500 Calories daily below calculated maintenance requirements. A weight loss of 10 to 20 pounds is generally recommended regardless of starting weight. Check with your physician or dietician.

▸ **Protein:** 10 to 20% of your calories should come from dietary protein. Certain diseases such as renal failure may reduce the recommended intake. Check with your physician.

▸ **Fat:** Less than 30% of your calories should come from fat.
Saturated fat: <10%. For cholesterol reduction <7%.
Polyunsaturated fat: <10%**Monounsaturated fat:** 10-15%

▸ **Cholesterol:** <300 mg/day. For cholesterol reduction < 200 mg/day.

▸ **Carbohydrates:** Obtain the remainder of your calories from this food group.
Sugar (sucrose): Sugar should be treated gram for gram like any other carbohydrate. *Diabetics can have their cake and eat it, too!*
Fructose: Fructose, especially naturally occurring is acceptable, as is its use in modest quantities for sweetening. However, large quantities should be avoided as it has been shown to increase LDL (bad) cholesterol.

▸ **Fiber:** 20-35 grams of combined soluble and insoluble fiber daily.

▸ **Sodium:** Recommendations vary between ≤2,400 mg and 3,000-mg daily consumption. If you have hypertension it is recommended that your intake be decreased to ≤2,000-mg daily.

▸ **Complications:** Underlying medical conditions may require your doctor to prescribe diets that vary from the above.

HOME BLOOD SUGAR MONITORING RECORDS

▶ Enter the times blood sugars were tested and the corresponding values.

▶ All home glucometers measure blood sugar from whole blood. However, some have been calibrated to give plasma values which run a little higher when compared to whole blood. It is therefore important for you to know which type of glucometer you have. Use the appropriate section for your glucometer to interpret your readings.

▶ Goal values (approximate) <u>**whole blood values**</u>:

   1. **Fasting =100 ± 20 mg/dL**. Usually first morning. No food or drink for ≥ 8 hours.

   2. **Before meals = 100 ± 20 mg/dL**. Essentially the same as fasting.

   3. **Bedtime = 120 ± 20 mg/dL**.

   4. **After meals = 140 mg/dL**. Two hours after meals. I found no data specifically addressing changes in this value.

▶ Goal values (approximate) <u>**plasma values**</u>:

   1. **Fasting =110 ± 20 mg/dL**. Usually first morning. No food or drink for ≥ 8 hours.

   2. **Before meals = 110 ± 20 mg/dL**. Essentially the same as fasting.

   3. **Bedtime = 130 ± 20 mg/dL**.

   4. **After meal = 150 mg/dL**. Two hours after meals. I found no data specifically addressing changes in this value.

▶ **Type 2 diabetics** should check their blood sugars daily if they are using insulin or sulfonurea medications (such as Amaryl, Glucotrol, Micronase, DiaBeta, Orinase, Tolinase or Diabinese). Measurements should be sufficiently frequent to optimally achieve glucose goals. Data have shown more frequent monitoring results in significantly lowered glycosylated hemoglobin levels. Type 2 diabetes is a progressive disease requiring frequent medication changes. My personal opinion is daily fasting and bedtime checks, at a minimum.

▶ **Type 1 diabetics** should check their sugars as prescribed by your physician to fit your insulin regimen. Generally, Type 1 diabetics should measure their blood sugars 3 or 4 times daily.

HOME BLOOD SUGAR MONITORING RECORDS

JANUARY

▸ Goal values (approximate) <u>whole blood values</u>:
1. **Fasting =100 ± 20 mg/dL.** Usually first morning. No food or drink for ≥ 8 hours.
2. **Before meals = 100 ± 20 mg/dL.** Essentially the same as fasting.
3. **Bedtime = 120 ± 20 mg/dL.**
4. **After meal = 140 mg/dL.** Two hours after meals.

▸ Goal values (approximate) <u>plasma values</u>:
1. **Fasting =110 ± 20 mg/dL.** Usually first morning. No food or drink for ≥ 8 hours.
2. **Before meals = 110 ± 20 mg/dL.** Essentially the same as fasting.
3. **Bedtime = 130 ± 20 mg/dL.**
4. **After meal = 150 mg/dL.** Two hours after meals.

Please fill in the following graph by placing an "X" in the appropriate box representing your blood sugar measured at the time of day indicated on the calendar. You may at your discretion connect the Xs with a line for easier viewing of your blood sugar levels.

January

Blood Sugar	Sunday				Monday				Tuesday			
	M	N	E	B	M	N	E	B	M	N	E	B
≥ 200												
190												
180												
170												
160												
150												
140												
130												
120												
110												
100												
90												
80												
70												
≤60												

M = Morning, N = Noon, E = Evening, B = Bedtime.

January

	Wednesday				Thursday 1				Friday 2				Saturday 3		
M	N	E	B	M	N	E	B	M	N	E	B	M	N	E	B

M = Morning, N = Noon, E = Evening, B = Bedtime.

January

Blood Sugar	Sunday 4				Monday 5				Tuesday 6			
	M	N	E	B	M	N	E	B	M	N	E	B
≥ 200												
190												
180												
170												
160												
150												
140												
130												
120												
110												
100												
90												
80												
70												
≤60												

M = Morning, N = Noon, E = Evening, B = Bedtime.

January

Wednesday 7				Thursday 8				Friday 9				Saturday 10			
M	N	E	B	M	N	E	B	M	N	E	B	M	N	E	B

M = Morning, N = Noon, E = Evening, B = Bedtime.

January

Blood Sugar	Sunday 11				Monday 12				Tuesday 13			
	M	N	E	B	M	N	E	B	M	N	E	B
≥ 200												
190												
180												
170												
160												
150												
140												
130												
120												
110												
100												
90												
80												
70												
≤60												

M = Morning, N = Noon, E = Evening, B = Bedtime.

January

Wednesday 14				Thursday 15				Friday 16				Saturday 17			
M	N	E	B	M	N	E	B	M	N	E	B	M	N	E	B

M = Morning, N = Noon, E = Evening, B = Bedtime.

January

Blood Sugar	Sunday 18				Monday 19				Tuesday 20			
	M	N	E	B	M	N	E	B	M	N	E	B
≥ 200												
190												
180												
170												
160												
150												
140												
130												
120												
110												
100												
90												
80												
70												
≤60												

M = Morning, N = Noon, E = Evening, B = Bedtime.

January

Wednesday 21				Thursday 22				Friday 23				Saturday 24			
M	N	E	B	M	N	E	B	M	N	E	B	M	N	E	B

M = Morning, N = Noon, E = Evening, B = Bedtime.

January

Blood Sugar	Sunday 25				Monday 26				Tuesday 27			
	M	N	E	B	M	N	E	B	M	N	E	B
≥ 200												
190												
180												
170												
160												
150												
140												
130												
120												
110												
100												
90												
80												
70												
≤60												

M = Morning, N = Noon, E = Evening, B = Bedtime.

January

Wednesday 28				Thursday 29				Friday 30				Saturday 31			
M	N	E	B	M	N	E	B	M	N	E	B	M	N	E	B

M = Morning, N = Noon, E = Evening, B = Bedtime.

HOME BLOOD SUGAR MONITORING RECORDS

FEBRUARY

▸ Goal values (approximate) <u>**whole blood values**</u>:
  1. **Fasting** =100 $\pm$ 20 **mg/dL**. Usually first morning. No food or drink for $\geq$ 8 hours.
  2. **Before meals** = 100 $\pm$ 20 **mg/dL**. Essentially the same as fasting.
  3. **Bedtime** = 120 $\pm$ 20 **mg/dL**.
  4. **After meal** = 140 **mg/dL**. Two hours after meals.

▸ Goal values (approximate) <u>**plasma values**</u>:
  1. **Fasting** =110 $\pm$ 20 **mg/dL**. Usually first morning. No food or drink for $\geq$ 8 hours.
  2. **Before meals** = 110 $\pm$ 20 **mg/dL**. Essentially the same as fasting.
  3. **Bedtime** = 130 $\pm$ 20 **mg/dL**.
  4. **After meal** = 150 **mg/dL**. Two hours after meals.

Please fill in the following graph by placing an "X" in the appropriate box representing your blood sugar measured at the time of day indicated on the calendar. You may at your discretion connect the Xs with a line for easier viewing of your blood sugar levels.

February

Blood Sugar	Sunday 1				Monday 2				Tuesday 3			
	M	N	E	B	M	N	E	B	M	N	E	B
≥ 200												
190												
180												
170												
160												
150												
140												
130												
120												
110												
100												
90												
80												
70												
≤60												

M = Morning, N = Noon, E = Evening, B = Bedtime.

February

Wednesday 4				Thursday 5				Friday 6				Saturday 7			
M	N	E	B	M	N	E	B	M	N	E	B	M	N	E	B

M = Morning, N = Noon, E = Evening, B = Bedtime.

February

Blood Sugar	Sunday 8				Monday 9				Tuesday 10			
	M	N	E	B	M	N	E	B	M	N	E	B
≥ 200												
190												
180												
170												
160												
150												
140												
130												
120												
110												
100												
90												
80												
70												
≤60												

M = Morning, N = Noon, E = Evening, B = Bedtime.

February

Wednesday 11				Thursday 12				Friday 13				Saturday 14			
M	N	E	B	M	N	E	B	M	N	E	B	M	N	E	B

M = Morning, N = Noon, E = Evening, B = Bedtime.

February

Blood Sugar	Sunday 15				Monday 16				Tuesday 17			
	M	N	E	B	M	N	E	B	M	N	E	B
≥ 200												
190												
180												
170												
160												
150												
140												
130												
120												
110												
100												
90												
80												
70												
≤60												

M = Morning, N = Noon, E = Evening, B = Bedtime.

February

Wednesday 18				Thursday 19				Friday 20				Saturday 21			
M	N	E	B	M	N	E	B	M	N	E	B	M	N	E	B

M = Morning, N = Noon, E = Evening, B = Bedtime.

February

Blood Sugar	Sunday 22				Monday 23				Tuesday 24			
	M	N	E	B	M	N	E	B	M	N	E	B
≥ 200												
190												
180												
170												
160												
150												
140												
130												
120												
110												
100												
90												
80												
70												
≤60												

M = Morning, N = Noon, E = Evening, B = Bedtime.

February

Wednesday 25				Thursday 26				Friday 27				Saturday 28			
M	N	E	B	M	N	E	B	M	N	E	B	M	N	E	B

M = Morning, N = Noon, E = Evening, B = Bedtime.

February

Blood Sugar	Sunday 29				Monday				Tuesday			
	M	N	E	B	M	N	E	B	M	N	E	B
≥ 200												
190												
180												
170												
160												
150												
140												
130												
120												
110												
100												
90												
80												
70												
≤60												

M = Morning, N = Noon, E = Evening, B = Bedtime.

February

Wednesday				Thursday				Friday				Saturday			
M	N	E	B	M	N	E	B	M	N	E	B	M	N	E	B

M = Morning, N = Noon, E = Evening, B = Bedtime.

HOME BLOOD SUGAR MONITORING RECORDS

MARCH

▶ Goal values (approximate) <u>whole blood values</u>:
1. **Fasting =100 ± 20 mg/dL.** Usually first morning. No food or drink for ≥ 8 hours.
2. **Before meals = 100 ± 20 mg/dL.** Essentially the same as fasting.
3. **Bedtime = 120 ± 20 mg/dL.**
4. **After meal = 140 mg/dL.** Two hours after meals.

▶ Goal values (approximate) <u>plasma values</u>:
1. **Fasting =110 ± 20 mg/dL.** Usually first morning. No food or drink for ≥ 8 hours.
2. **Before meals = 110 ± 20 mg/dL.** Essentially the same as fasting.
3. **Bedtime = 130 ± 20 mg/dL.**
4. **After meal = 150 mg/dL.** Two hours after meals.

Please fill in the following graph by placing an "X" in the appropriate box representing your blood sugar measured at the time of day indicated on the calendar. You may at your discretion connect the Xs with a line for easier viewing of your blood sugar levels.

March

Blood Sugar	Sunday				Monday 1				Tuesday 2			
	M	N	E	B	M	N	E	B	M	N	E	B
≥ 200												
190												
180												
170												
160												
150												
140												
130												
120												
110												
100												
90												
80												
70												
≤60												

M = Morning, N = Noon, E = Evening, B = Bedtime.

March

Wednesday 3				Thursday 4				Friday 5				Saturday 6			
M	N	E	B	M	N	E	B	M	N	E	B	M	N	E	B

M = Morning, N = Noon, E = Evening, B = Bedtime.

March

Blood Sugar	Sunday 7				Monday 8				Tuesday 9			
	M	N	E	B	M	N	E	B	M	N	E	B
≥ 200												
190												
180												
170												
160												
150												
140												
130												
120												
110												
100												
90												
80												
70												
≤60												

M = Morning, N = Noon, E = Evening, B = Bedtime.

March

Wednesday 10				Thursday 11				Friday 12				Saturday 13			
M	N	E	B	M	N	E	B	M	N	E	B	M	N	E	B

M = Morning, N = Noon, E = Evening, B = Bedtime.

March

Blood Sugar	Sunday 14				Monday 15				Tuesday 16			
	M	N	E	B	M	N	E	B	M	N	E	B
≥ 200												
190												
180												
170												
160												
150												
140												
130												
120												
110												
100												
90												
80												
70												
≤60												

M = Morning, N = Noon, E = Evening, B = Bedtime.

March

Wednesday 17				Thursday 18				Friday 19				Saturday 20			
M	N	E	B	M	N	E	B	M	N	E	B	M	N	E	B

M = Morning, N = Noon, E = Evening, B = Bedtime.

March

Blood Sugar	Sunday 21				Monday 22				Tuesday 23			
	M	N	E	B	M	N	E	B	M	N	E	B
≥ 200												
190												
180												
170												
160												
150												
140												
130												
120												
110												
100												
90												
80												
70												
≤60												

M = Morning, N = Noon, E = Evening, B = Bedtime.

March

Wednesday 24				Thursday 25				Friday 26				Saturday 27			
M	N	E	B	M	N	E	B	M	N	E	B	M	N	E	B

M = Morning, N = Noon, E = Evening, B = Bedtime.

March

Blood Sugar	Sunday 28				Monday 29				Tuesday 30			
	M	N	E	B	M	N	E	B	M	N	E	B
≥ 200												
190												
180												
170												
160												
150												
140												
130												
120												
110												
100												
90												
80												
70												
≤60												

M = Morning, N = Noon, E = Evening, B = Bedtime.

March

Wednesday 31				Thursday				Friday				Saturday			
M	N	E	B	M	N	E	B	M	N	E	B	M	N	E	B

M = Morning, N = Noon, E = Evening, B = Bedtime.

HOME BLOOD SUGAR MONITORING RECORDS

APRIL

▸ Goal values (approximate) <u>**whole blood values**</u>:
1. **Fasting =100 ± 20 mg/dL.** Usually first morning. No food or drink for ≥ 8 hours.
2. **Before meals = 100 ± 20 mg/dL.** Essentially the same as fasting.
3. **Bedtime = 120 ± 20 mg/dL.**
4. **After meal = 140 mg/dL.** Two hours after meals.

▸ Goal values (approximate) <u>**plasma values**</u>:
1. **Fasting =110 ± 20 mg/dL.** Usually first morning. No food or drink for ≥ 8 hours.
2. **Before meals = 110 ± 20 mg/dL.** Essentially the same as fasting.
3. **Bedtime = 130 ± 20 mg/dL.**
4. **After meal = 150 mg/dL.** Two hours after meals.

Please fill in the following graph by placing an "X" in the appropriate box representing your blood sugar measured at the time of day indicated on the calendar. You may at your discretion connect the Xs with a line for easier viewing of your blood sugar levels.

April

Blood Sugar	Sunday				Monday				Tuesday			
	M	N	E	B	M	N	E	B	M	N	E	B
≥ 200												
190												
180												
170												
160												
150												
140												
130												
120												
110												
100												
90												
80												
70												
≤60												

M = Morning, N = Noon, E = Evening, B = Bedtime.

April

Wednesday				Thursday 1				Friday 2				Saturday 3			
M	N	E	B	M	N	E	B	M	N	E	B	M	N	E	B

M = Morning, N = Noon, E = Evening, B = Bedtime.

April

Blood Sugar	Sunday 4				Monday 5				Tuesday 6			
	M	N	E	B	M	N	E	B	M	N	E	B
≥ 200												
190												
180												
170												
160												
150												
140												
130												
120												
110												
100												
90												
80												
70												
≤60												

M = Morning, N = Noon, E = Evening, B = Bedtime.

April

Wednesday 7				Thursday 8				Friday 9				Saturday 10			
M	N	E	B	M	N	E	B	M	N	E	B	M	N	E	B

M = Morning, N = Noon, E = Evening, B = Bedtime.

April

Blood Sugar	Sunday 11				Monday 12				Tuesday 13			
	M	N	E	B	M	N	E	B	M	N	E	B
≥ 200												
190												
180												
170												
160												
150												
140												
130												
120												
110												
100												
90												
80												
70												
≤60												

M = Morning, N = Noon, E = Evening, B = Bedtime.

April

Wednesday 14				Thursday 15				Friday 16				Saturday 17			
M	N	E	B	M	N	E	B	M	N	E	B	M	N	E	B

M = Morning, N = Noon, E = Evening, B = Bedtime.

April

Blood Sugar	Sunday 18				Monday 19				Tuesday 20			
	M	N	E	B	M	N	E	B	M	N	E	B
≥ 200												
190												
180												
170												
160												
150												
140												
130												
120												
110												
100												
90												
80												
70												
≤60												

M = Morning, N = Noon, E = Evening, B = Bedtime.

April

Wednesday 21				Thursday 22				Friday 23				Saturday 24			
M	N	E	B	M	N	E	B	M	N	E	B	M	N	E	B

M = Morning, N = Noon, E = Evening, B = Bedtime.

April

Blood Sugar	Sunday 25				Monday 26				Tuesday 27			
	M	N	E	B	M	N	E	B	M	N	E	B
≥ 200												
190												
180												
170												
160												
150												
140												
130												
120												
110												
100												
90												
80												
70												
≤60												

M = Morning, N = Noon, E = Evening, B = Bedtime.

April

Wednesday 28				Thursday 29				Friday 30				Saturday			
M	N	E	B	M	N	E	B	M	N	E	B	M	N	E	B

M = Morning, N = Noon, E = Evening, B = Bedtime.

HOME BLOOD SUGAR MONITORING RECORDS

May

▸ Goal values (approximate) <u>whole blood values</u>:
1. **Fasting =100 ± 20 mg/dL.** Usually first morning. No food or drink for ≥ 8 hours.
2. **Before meals = 100 ± 20 mg/dL.** Essentially the same as fasting.
3. **Bedtime = 120 ± 20 mg/dL.**
4. **After meal = 140 mg/dL.** Two hours after meals.

▸ Goal values (approximate) <u>plasma values</u>:
1. **Fasting =110 ± 20 mg/dL.** Usually first morning. No food or drink for ≥ 8 hours.
2. **Before meals = 110 ± 20 mg/dL.** Essentially the same as fasting.
3. **Bedtime = 130 ± 20 mg/dL.**
4. **After meal = 150 mg/dL.** Two hours after meals.

Please fill in the following graph by placing an "X" in the appropriate box representing your blood sugar measured at the time of day indicated on the calendar. You may at your discretion connect the Xs with a line for easier viewing of your blood sugar levels.

May

Blood Sugar	Sunday				Monday				Tuesday			
	M	N	E	B	M	N	E	B	M	N	E	B
≥ 200												
190												
180												
170												
160												
150												
140												
130												
120												
110												
100												
90												
80												
70												
≤60												

M = Morning, N = Noon, E = Evening, B = Bedtime.

May

Wednesday				Thursday				Friday				Saturday 1			
M	N	E	B	M	N	E	B	M	N	E	B	M	N	E	B

M = Morning, N = Noon, E = Evening, B = Bedtime.

May

Blood Sugar	Sunday 2				Monday 3				Tuesday 4			
	M	N	E	B	M	N	E	B	M	N	E	B
≥ 200												
190												
180												
170												
160												
150												
140												
130												
120												
110												
100												
90												
80												
70												
≤60												

M = Morning, N = Noon, E = Evening, B = Bedtime.

May

Wednesday 5				Thursday 6				Friday 7				Saturday 8			
M	N	E	B	M	N	E	B	M	N	E	B	M	N	E	B

M = Morning, N = Noon, E = Evening, B = Bedtime.

May

Blood Sugar	Sunday 9				Monday 10				Tuesday 11			
	M	N	E	B	M	N	E	B	M	N	E	B
≥ 200												
190												
180												
170												
160												
150												
140												
130												
120												
110												
100												
90												
80												
70												
≤60												

M = Morning, N = Noon, E = Evening, B = Bedtime.

May

Wednesday 12				Thursday 13				Friday 14				Saturday 15			
M	N	E	B	M	N	E	B	M	N	E	B	M	N	E	B

M = Morning, N = Noon, E = Evening, B = Bedtime.

May

Blood Sugar	Sunday 16				Monday 17				Tuesday 18			
	M	N	E	B	M	N	E	B	M	N	E	B
≥ 200												
190												
180												
170												
160												
150												
140												
130												
120												
110												
100												
90												
80												
70												
≤60												

M = Morning, N = Noon, E = Evening, B = Bedtime.

May

Wednesday 19				Thursday 20				Friday 21				Saturday 22			
M	N	E	B	M	N	E	B	M	N	E	B	M	N	E	B

M = Morning, N = Noon, E = Evening, B = Bedtime.

May

Blood Sugar	Sunday 23				Monday 24				Tuesday 25			
	M	N	E	B	M	N	E	B	M	N	E	B
≥ 200												
190												
180												
170												
160												
150												
140												
130												
120												
110												
100												
90												
80												
70												
≤60												

M = Morning, N = Noon, E = Evening, B = Bedtime.

May

Wednesday 26				Thursday 27				Friday 28				Saturday 29			
M	N	E	B	M	N	E	B	M	N	E	B	M	N	E	B

M = Morning, N = Noon, E = Evening, B = Bedtime.

May

Blood Sugar	Sunday 30				Monday 31				Tuesday			
	M	N	E	B	M	N	E	B	M	N	E	B
≥ 200												
190												
180												
170												
160												
150												
140												
130												
120												
110												
100												
90												
80												
70												
≤60												

M = Morning, N = Noon, E = Evening, B = Bedtime.

May

Wednesday				Thursday				Friday				Saturday			
M	N	E	B	M	N	E	B	M	N	E	B	M	N	E	B

M = Morning, N = Noon, E = Evening, B = Bedtime.

HOME BLOOD SUGAR MONITORING RECORDS

June

▶ Goal values (approximate) <u>**whole blood values**</u>:
1. **Fasting** =100 ± 20 **mg/dL.** Usually first morning. No food or drink for ≥ 8 hours.
2. **Before meals** = 100 ± 20 **mg/dL.** Essentially the same as fasting.
3. **Bedtime** = 120 ± 20 **mg/dL.**
4. **After meal** = 140 **mg/dL.** Two hours after meals.

▶ Goal values (approximate) <u>**plasma values**</u>:
1. **Fasting** =110 ± 20 **mg/dL.** Usually first morning. No food or drink for ≥ 8 hours.
2. **Before meals** = 110 ± 20 **mg/dL.** Essentially the same as fasting.
3. **Bedtime** = 130 ± 20 **mg/dL.**
4. **After meal** = 150 **mg/dL.** Two hours after meals.

Please fill in the following graph by placing an "X" in the appropriate box representing your blood sugar measured at the time of day indicated on the calendar. You may at your discretion connect the Xs with a line for easier viewing of your blood sugar levels.

June

Blood Sugar	Sunday				Monday				Tuesday 1			
	M	N	E	B	M	N	E	B	M	N	E	B
≥ 200												
190												
180												
170												
160												
150												
140												
130												
120												
110												
100												
90												
80												
70												
≤60												

M = Morning, N = Noon, E = Evening, B = Bedtime.

June

Wednesday 2				Thursday 3				Friday 4				Saturday 5			
M	N	E	B	M	N	E	B	M	N	E	B	M	N	E	B

M = Morning, N = Noon, E = Evening, B = Bedtime.

June

Blood Sugar	Sunday 6				Monday 7				Tuesday 8			
	M	N	E	B	M	N	E	B	M	N	E	B
≥ 200												
190												
180												
170												
160												
150												
140												
130												
120												
110												
100												
90												
80												
70												
≤60												

M = Morning, N = Noon, E = Evening, B = Bedtime.

June

Wednesday 9				Thursday 10				Friday 11				Saturday 12			
M	N	E	B	M	N	E	B	M	N	E	B	M	N	E	B

M = Morning, N = Noon, E = Evening, B = Bedtime.

June

Blood Sugar	Sunday 13				Monday 14				Tuesday 15			
	M	N	E	B	M	N	E	B	M	N	E	B
≥ 200												
190												
180												
170												
160												
150												
140												
130												
120												
110												
100												
90												
80												
70												
≤60												

M = Morning, N = Noon, E = Evening, B = Bedtime.

June

Wednesday 16				Thursday 17				Friday 18				Saturday 19			
M	N	E	B	M	N	E	B	M	N	E	B	M	N	E	B

M = Morning, N = Noon, E = Evening, B = Bedtime.

June

Blood Sugar	Sunday 20				Monday 21				Tuesday 22			
	M	N	E	B	M	N	E	B	M	N	E	B
≥ 200												
190												
180												
170												
160												
150												
140												
130												
120												
110												
100												
90												
80												
70												
≤60												

M = Morning, N = Noon, E = Evening, B = Bedtime.

June

Wednesday 23				Thursday 24				Friday 25				Saturday 26			
M	N	E	B	M	N	E	B	M	N	E	B	M	N	E	B

M = Morning, N = Noon, E = Evening, B = Bedtime.

June

Blood Sugar	Sunday 27				Monday 28				Tuesday 29			
	M	N	E	B	M	N	E	B	M	N	E	B
≥ 200												
190												
180												
170												
160												
150												
140												
130												
120												
110												
100												
90												
80												
70												
≤60												

M = Morning, N = Noon, E = Evening, B = Bedtime.

June

Wednesday 30				Thursday				Friday				Saturday			
M	N	E	B	M	N	E	B	M	N	E	B	M	N	E	B

M = Morning, N = Noon, E = Evening, B = Bedtime.

HOME BLOOD SUGAR MONITORING RECORDS

July

▶ Goal values (approximate) <u>whole blood values</u>:

1. **Fasting** =100 ± 20 mg/dL. Usually first morning. No food or drink for ≥ 8 hours.
2. **Before meals** = 100 ± 20 mg/dL. Essentially the same as fasting.
3. **Bedtime** = 120 ± 20 mg/dL.
4. **After meal** = 140 mg/dL. Two hours after meals.

▶ Goal values (approximate) <u>plasma values</u>:

1. **Fasting** =110 ± 20 mg/dL. Usually first morning. No food or drink for ≥ 8 hours.
2. **Before meals** = 110 ± 20 mg/dL. Essentially the same as fasting.
3. **Bedtime** = 130 ± 20 mg/dL.
4. **After meal** = 150 mg/dL. Two hours after meals.

Please fill in the following graph by placing an "X" in the appropriate box representing your blood sugar measured at the time of day indicated on the calendar. You may at your discretion connect the Xs with a line for easier viewing of your blood sugar levels.

July

Blood Sugar	Sunday				Monday				Tuesday			
	M	N	E	B	M	N	E	B	M	N	E	B
≥ 200												
190												
180												
170												
160												
150												
140												
130												
120												
110												
100												
90												
80												
70												
≤60												

M = Morning, N = Noon, E = Evening, B = Bedtime.

July

Wednesday				Thursday 1				Friday 2				Saturday 3			
M	N	E	B	M	N	E	B	M	N	E	B	M	N	E	B

M = Morning, N = Noon, E = Evening, B = Bedtime.

July

Blood Sugar	Sunday 4				Monday 5				Tuesday 6			
	M	N	E	B	M	N	E	B	M	N	E	B
≥ 200												
190												
180												
170												
160												
150												
140												
130												
120												
110												
100												
90												
80												
70												
≤60												

M = Morning, N = Noon, E = Evening, B = Bedtime.

July

Wednesday 7				Thursday 8				Friday 9				Saturday 10			
M	N	E	B	M	N	E	B	M	N	E	B	M	N	E	B

M = Morning, N = Noon, E = Evening, B = Bedtime.

July

Blood Sugar	Sunday 11				Monday 12				Tuesday 13			
	M	N	E	B	M	N	E	B	M	N	E	B
≥ 200												
190												
180												
170												
160												
150												
140												
130												
120												
110												
100												
90												
80												
70												
≤60												

M = Morning, N = Noon, E = Evening, B = Bedtime.

July

Wednesday 14				Thursday 15				Friday 16				Saturday 17			
M	N	E	B	M	N	E	B	M	N	E	B	M	N	E	B

M = Morning, N = Noon, E = Evening, B = Bedtime.

July

Blood Sugar	Sunday 18				Monday 19				Tuesday 20			
	M	N	E	B	M	N	E	B	M	N	E	B
≥ 200												
190												
180												
170												
160												
150												
140												
130												
120												
110												
100												
90												
80												
70												
≤60												

M = Morning, N = Noon, E = Evening, B = Bedtime.

July

Wednesday 21				Thursday 22				Friday 23				Saturday 24			
M	N	E	B	M	N	E	B	M	N	E	B	M	N	E	B

M = Morning, N = Noon, E = Evening, B = Bedtime.

July

Blood Sugar	Sunday 25				Monday 26				Tuesday 27			
	M	N	E	B	M	N	E	B	M	N	E	B
≥ 200												
190												
180												
170												
160												
150												
140												
130												
120												
110												
100												
90												
80												
70												
≤60												

M = Morning, N = Noon, E = Evening, B = Bedtime.

July

Wednesday 28				Thursday 29				Friday 30				Saturday 31			
M	N	E	B	M	N	E	B	M	N	E	B	M	N	E	B

M = Morning, N = Noon, E = Evening, B = Bedtime.

HOME BLOOD SUGAR MONITORING RECORDS

August

▶ Goal values (approximate) <u>**whole blood values**</u>:
   1. **Fasting** =100 ± 20 **mg/dL.** Usually first morning. No food or drink for ≥ 8 hours.
   2. **Before meals** = 100 ± 20 **mg/dL.** Essentially the same as fasting.
   3. **Bedtime** = 120 ± 20 **mg/dL.**
   4. **After meal** = 140 **mg/dL.** Two hours after meals.

▶ Goal values (approximate) <u>**plasma values**</u>:
   1. **Fasting** =110 ± 20 **mg/dL.** Usually first morning. No food or drink for ≥ 8 hours.
   2. **Before meals** = 110 ± 20 **mg/dL.** Essentially the same as fasting.
   3. **Bedtime** = 130 ± 20 **mg/dL.**
   4. **After meal** = 150 **mg/dL.** Two hours after meals.

Please fill in the following graph by placing an "X" in the appropriate box representing your blood sugar measured at the time of day indicated on the calendar. You may at your discretion connect the Xs with a line for easier viewing of your blood sugar levels.

August

Blood Sugar	Sunday 1				Monday 2				Tuesday 3			
	M	N	E	B	M	N	E	B	M	N	E	B
≥ 200												
190												
180												
170												
160												
150												
140												
130												
120												
110												
100												
90												
80												
70												
≤60												

M = Morning, N = Noon, E = Evening, B = Bedtime.

August

Wednesday 4				Thursday 5				Friday 6				Saturday 7			
M	N	E	B	M	N	E	B	M	N	E	B	M	N	E	B

M = Morning, N = Noon, E = Evening, B = Bedtime.

August

Blood Sugar	Sunday 8				Monday 9				Tuesday 10			
	M	N	E	B	M	N	E	B	M	N	E	B
≥ 200												
190												
180												
170												
160												
150												
140												
130												
120												
110												
100												
90												
80												
70												
≤60												

M = Morning, N = Noon, E = Evening, B = Bedtime.

August

Wednesday 11				Thursday 12				Friday 13				Saturday 14			
M	N	E	B	M	N	E	B	M	N	E	B	M	N	E	B

M = Morning, N = Noon, E = Evening, B = Bedtime.

August

Blood Sugar	Sunday 15				Monday 16				Tuesday 17			
	M	N	E	B	M	N	E	B	M	N	E	B
≥ 200												
190												
180												
170												
160												
150												
140												
130												
120												
110												
100												
90												
80												
70												
≤60												

M = Morning, N = Noon, E = Evening, B = Bedtime.

August

Wednesday 18				Thursday 19				Friday 20				Saturday 21			
M	N	E	B	M	N	E	B	M	N	E	B	M	N	E	B

M = Morning, N = Noon, E = Evening, B = Bedtime.

August

Blood Sugar	Sunday 22				Monday 23				Tuesday 24			
	M	N	E	B	M	N	E	B	M	N	E	B
≥ 200												
190												
180												
170												
160												
150												
140												
130												
120												
110												
100												
90												
80												
70												
≤60												

M = Morning, N = Noon, E = Evening, B = Bedtime.

August

Wednesday 25				Thursday 26				Friday 27				Saturday 28			
M	N	E	B	M	N	E	B	M	N	E	B	M	N	E	B

M = Morning, N = Noon, E = Evening, B = Bedtime.

August

Blood Sugar	Sunday 29				Monday 30				Tuesday 31			
	M	N	E	B	M	N	E	B	M	N	E	B
≥ 200												
190												
180												
170												
160												
150												
140												
130												
120												
110												
100												
90												
80												
70												
≤60												

M = Morning, N = Noon, E = Evening, B = Bedtime.

August

Wednesday				Thursday				Friday				Saturday			
M	N	E	B	M	N	E	B	M	N	E	B	M	N	E	B

M = Morning, N = Noon, E = Evening, B = Bedtime.

HOME BLOOD SUGAR MONITORING RECORDS

September

▶ Goal values (approximate) <u>**whole blood values**</u>:
  1. **Fasting** =100 ± 20 **mg/dL**. Usually first morning. No food or drink for ≥ 8 hours.
  2. **Before meals** = 100 ± 20 **mg/dL**. Essentially the same as fasting.
  3. **Bedtime** = 120 ± 20 **mg/dL**.
  4. **After meal** = 140 **mg/dL**. Two hours after meals.

▶ Goal values (approximate) <u>**plasma values**</u>:
  1. **Fasting** =110 ± 20 **mg/dL**. Usually first morning. No food or drink for ≥ 8 hours.
  2. **Before meals** = 110 ± 20 **mg/dL**. Essentially the same as fasting.
  3. **Bedtime** = 130 ± 20 **mg/dL**.
  4. **After meal** = 150 **mg/dL**. Two hours after meals.

Please fill in the following graph by placing an "X" in the appropriate box representing your blood sugar measured at the time of day indicated on the calendar. You may at your discretion connect the Xs with a line for easier viewing of your blood sugar levels.

September

Blood Sugar	Sunday				Monday				Tuesday			
	M	N	E	B	M	N	E	B	M	N	E	B
≥ 200												
190												
180												
170												
160												
150												
140												
130												
120												
110												
100												
90												
80												
70												
≤60												

M = Morning, N = Noon, E = Evening, B = Bedtime.

September

Wednesday 1				Thursday 2				Friday 3				Saturday 4			
M	N	E	B	M	N	E	B	M	N	E	B	M	N	E	B

M = Morning, N = Noon, E = Evening, B = Bedtime.

September

Blood Sugar	Sunday 5				Monday 6				Tuesday 7			
	M	N	E	B	M	N	E	B	M	N	E	B
≥ 200												
190												
180												
170												
160												
150												
140												
130												
120												
110												
100												
90												
80												
70												
≤60												

M = Morning, N = Noon, E = Evening, B = Bedtime.

September

Wednesday 8				Thursday 9				Friday 10				Saturday 11			
M	N	E	B	M	N	E	B	M	N	E	B	M	N	E	B

M = Morning, N = Noon, E = Evening, B = Bedtime.

September

Blood Sugar	Sunday 12				Monday 13				Tuesday 14			
	M	N	E	B	M	N	E	B	M	N	E	B
≥ 200												
190												
180												
170												
160												
150												
140												
130												
120												
110												
100												
90												
80												
70												
≤60												

M = Morning, N = Noon, E = Evening, B = Bedtime.

September

Wednesday 15				Thursday 16				Friday 17				Saturday 18			
M	N	E	B	M	N	E	B	M	N	E	B	M	N	E	B

M = Morning, N = Noon, E = Evening, B = Bedtime.

September

Blood Sugar	Sunday 19				Monday 20				Tuesday 21			
	M	N	E	B	M	N	E	B	M	N	E	B
≥ 200												
190												
180												
170												
160												
150												
140												
130												
120												
110												
100												
90												
80												
70												
≤60												

M = Morning, N = Noon, E = Evening, B = Bedtime.

September

Wednesday 22				Thursday 23				Friday 24				Saturday 25			
M	N	E	B	M	N	E	B	M	N	E	B	M	N	E	B

M = Morning, N = Noon, E = Evening, B = Bedtime.

September

Blood Sugar	Sunday 26				Monday 27				Tuesday 28			
	M	N	E	B	M	N	E	B	M	N	E	B
≥ 200												
190												
180												
170												
160												
150												
140												
130												
120												
110												
100												
90												
80												
70												
≤60												

M = Morning, N = Noon, E = Evening, B = Bedtime.

September

Wednesday 29				Thursday 30				Friday				Saturday			
M	N	E	B	M	N	E	B	M	N	E	B	M	N	E	B

M = Morning, N = Noon, E = Evening, B = Bedtime.

HOME BLOOD SUGAR MONITORING RECORDS

October

▸ Goal values (approximate) <u>**whole blood values**</u>:
  1. **Fasting** =100 ± 20 mg/dL. Usually first morning. No food or drink for ≥ 8 hours.
  2. **Before meals** = 100 ± 20 mg/dL. Essentially the same as fasting.
  3. **Bedtime** = 120 ± 20 mg/dL.
  4. **After meal** = 140 mg/dL. Two hours after meals.

▸ Goal values (approximate) <u>**plasma values**</u>:
  1. **Fasting** =110 ± 20 mg/dL. Usually first morning. No food or drink for ≥ 8 hours.
  2. **Before meals** = 110 ± 20 mg/dL. Essentially the same as fasting.
  3. **Bedtime** = 130 ± 20 mg/dL.
  4. **After meal** = 150 mg/dL. Two hours after meals.

Please fill in the following graph by placing an "X" in the appropriate box representing your blood sugar measured at the time of day indicated on the calendar. You may at your discretion connect the Xs with a line for easier viewing of your blood sugar levels.

October

Blood Sugar	Sunday				Monday				Tuesday			
	M	N	E	B	M	N	E	B	M	N	E	B
≥ 200												
190												
180												
170												
160												
150												
140												
130												
120												
110												
100												
90												
80												
70												
≤60												

M = Morning, N = Noon, E = Evening, B = Bedtime.

October

Wednesday				Thursday				Friday 1				Saturday 2			
M	N	E	B	M	N	E	B	M	N	E	B	M	N	E	B

M = Morning, N = Noon, E = Evening, B = Bedtime.

October

Blood Sugar	Sunday 3				Monday 4				Tuesday 5			
	M	N	E	B	M	N	E	B	M	N	E	B
≥ 200												
190												
180												
170												
160												
150												
140												
130												
120												
110												
100												
90												
80												
70												
≤60												

M = Morning, N = Noon, E = Evening, B = Bedtime.

October

Wednesday 6				Thursday 7				Friday 8				Saturday 9			
M	N	E	B	M	N	E	B	M	N	E	B	M	N	E	B

M = Morning, N = Noon, E = Evening, B = Bedtime.

October

Blood Sugar	Sunday 10				Monday 11				Tuesday 12			
	M	N	E	B	M	N	E	B	M	N	E	B
≥ 200												
190												
180												
170												
160												
150												
140												
130												
120												
110												
100												
90												
80												
70												
≤60												

M = Morning, N = Noon, E = Evening, B = Bedtime.

October

Wednesday 13				Thursday 14				Friday 15				Saturday 16			
M	N	E	B	M	N	E	B	M	N	E	B	M	N	E	B

M = Morning, N = Noon, E = Evening, B = Bedtime.

October

Blood Sugar	Sunday 17				Monday 18				Tuesday 19			
	M	N	E	B	M	N	E	B	M	N	E	B
≥ 200												
190												
180												
170												
160												
150												
140												
130												
120												
110												
100												
90												
80												
70												
≤60												

M = Morning, N = Noon, E = Evening, B = Bedtime.

October

Wednesday 20				Thursday 21				Friday 22				Saturday 23			
M	N	E	B	M	N	E	B	M	N	E	B	M	N	E	B

M = Morning, N = Noon, E = Evening, B = Bedtime.

October

Blood Sugar	Sunday 24				Monday 25				Tuesday 26			
	M	N	E	B	M	N	E	B	M	N	E	B
≥ 200												
190												
180												
170												
160												
150												
140												
130												
120												
110												
100												
90												
80												
70												
≤60												

M = Morning, N = Noon, E = Evening, B = Bedtime.

October

Wednesday 27				Thursday 28				Friday 29				Saturday 30			
M	N	E	B	M	N	E	B	M	N	E	B	M	N	E	B

M = Morning, N = Noon, E = Evening, B = Bedtime.

October

Blood Sugar	Sunday 31				Monday				Tuesday			
	M	N	E	B	M	N	E	B	M	N	E	B
≥ 200												
190												
180												
170												
160												
150												
140												
130												
120												
110												
100												
90												
80												
70												
≤60												

M = Morning, N = Noon, E = Evening, B = Bedtime.

October

Wednesday				Thursday				Friday				Saturday			
M	N	E	B	M	N	E	B	M	N	E	B	M	N	E	B

M = Morning, N = Noon, E = Evening, B = Bedtime.

HOME BLOOD SUGAR MONITORING RECORDS

November

▶ Goal values (approximate) <u>**whole blood values**</u>:
  1. **Fasting =100 ± 20 mg/dL.** Usually first morning. No food or drink for ≥ 8 hours.
  2. **Before meals = 100 ± 20 mg/dL.** Essentially the same as fasting.
  3. **Bedtime = 120 ± 20 mg/dL.**
  4. **After meal = 140 mg/dL.** Two hours after meals.

▶ Goal values (approximate) <u>**plasma values**</u>:
  1. **Fasting =110 ± 20 mg/dL.** Usually first morning. No food or drink for ≥ 8 hours.
  2. **Before meals = 110 ± 20 mg/dL.** Essentially the same as fasting.
  3. **Bedtime = 130 ± 20 mg/dL.**
  4. **After meal = 150 mg/dL.** Two hours after meals.

Please fill in the following graph by placing an "X" in the appropriate box representing your blood sugar measured at the time of day indicated on the calendar. You may at your discretion connect the Xs with a line for easier viewing of your blood sugar levels.

November

Blood Sugar	Sunday				Monday 1				Tuesday 2			
	M	N	E	B	M	N	E	B	M	N	E	B
≥ 200												
190												
180												
170												
160												
150												
140												
130												
120												
110												
100												
90												
80												
70												
≤60												

M = Morning, N = Noon, E = Evening, B = Bedtime.

November

Wednesday 3				Thursday 4				Friday 5				Saturday 6			
M	N	E	B	M	N	E	B	M	N	E	B	M	N	E	B

M = Morning, N = Noon, E = Evening, B = Bedtime.

Its time to order your new *DIABETIC DIARY 2005!* 1-877-823-9235

Notes:

November

Blood Sugar	Sunday 7				Monday 8				Tuesday 9			
	M	N	E	B	M	N	E	B	M	N	E	B
≥ 200												
190												
180												
170												
160												
150												
140												
130												
120												
110												
100												
90												
80												
70												
≤60												

M = Morning, N = Noon, E = Evening, B = Bedtime.

November

Wednesday 10				Thursday 11				Friday 12				Saturday 13			
M	N	E	B	M	N	E	B	M	N	E	B	M	N	E	B

M = Morning, N = Noon, E = Evening, B = Bedtime.

Its time to order your new *DIABETIC DIARY 2005!* 1-877-823-9235

Notes:

November

Blood Sugar	Sunday 14				Monday 15				Tuesday 16			
	M	N	E	B	M	N	E	B	M	N	E	B
≥ 200												
190												
180												
170												
160												
150												
140												
130												
120												
110												
100												
90												
80												
70												
≤60												

M = Morning, N = Noon, E = Evening, B = Bedtime.

November

Wednesday 17				Thursday 18				Friday 19				Saturday 20			
M	N	E	B	M	N	E	B	M	N	E	B	M	N	E	B

M = Morning, N = Noon, E = Evening, B = Bedtime.

Its time to order your new *DIABETIC DIARY 2005!* 1-877-823-9235

Notes:

November

Blood Sugar	Sunday 21				Monday 22				Tuesday 23			
	M	N	E	B	M	N	E	B	M	N	E	B
≥ 200												
190												
180												
170												
160												
150												
140												
130												
120												
110												
100												
90												
80												
70												
≤60												

M = Morning, N = Noon, E = Evening, B = Bedtime.

November

Wednesday 24				Thursday 25				Friday 26				Saturday 27			
M	N	E	B	M	N	E	B	M	N	E	B	M	N	E	B

M = Morning, N = Noon, E = Evening, B = Bedtime.

Its time to order your new *DIABETIC DIARY 2005!* 1-877-823-9235

Notes:

November

Blood Sugar	Sunday 28				Monday 29				Tuesday 30			
	M	N	E	B	M	N	E	B	M	N	E	B
≥ 200												
190												
180												
170												
160												
150												
140												
130												
120												
110												
100												
90												
80												
70												
≤60												

M = Morning, N = Noon, E = Evening, B = Bedtime.

November

Wednesday				Thursday				Friday				Saturday			
M	N	E	B	M	N	E	B	M	N	E	B	M	N	E	B

M = Morning, N = Noon, E = Evening, B = Bedtime.

Its time to order your new *DIABETIC DIARY 2005!* 1-877-823-9235

Notes:

HOME BLOOD SUGAR MONITORING RECORDS

December

▸ Goal values (approximate) <u>whole blood values</u>:
1. **Fasting =100 ± 20 mg/dL.** Usually first morning. No food or drink for ≥ 8 hours.
2. **Before meals = 100 ± 20 mg/dL.** Essentially the same as fasting.
3. **Bedtime = 120 ± 20 mg/dL.**
4. **After meal = 140 mg/dL.** Two hours after meals.

▸ Goal values (approximate) <u>plasma values</u>:
1. **Fasting =110 ± 20 mg/dL.** Usually first morning. No food or drink for ≥ 8 hours.
2. **Before meals = 110 ± 20 mg/dL.** Essentially the same as fasting.
3. **Bedtime = 130 ± 20 mg/dL.**
4. **After meal = 150 mg/dL.** Two hours after meals.

Please fill in the following graph by placing an "X" in the appropriate box representing 0your blood sugar measured at the time of day indicated on the calendar. You may at your discretion connect the Xs with a line for easier viewing of your blood sugar levels.

December

Blood Sugar	Sunday				Monday				Tuesday			
	M	N	E	B	M	N	E	B	M	N	E	B
≥ 200												
190												
180												
170												
160												
150												
140												
130												
120												
110												
100												
90												
80												
70												
≤60												

M = Morning, N = Noon, E = Evening, B = Bedtime.

December

Wednesday 1				Thursday 2				Friday 3				Saturday 4			
M	N	E	B	M	N	E	B	M	N	E	B	M	N	E	B

M = Morning, N = Noon, E = Evening, B = Bedtime.

Its time to order your new *DIABETIC DIARY 2005!* 1-877-823-9235

Notes:

December

Blood Sugar	Sunday 5				Monday 6				Tuesday 7			
	M	N	E	B	M	N	E	B	M	N	E	B
≥ 200												
190												
180												
170												
160												
150												
140												
130												
120												
110												
100												
90												
80												
70												
≤60												

M = Morning, N = Noon, E = Evening, B = Bedtime.

December

Wednesday 8				Thursday 9				Friday 10				Saturday 11			
M	N	E	B	M	N	E	B	M	N	E	B	M	N	E	B

M = Morning, N = Noon, E = Evening, B = Bedtime.

Its time to order your new *DIABETIC DIARY 2005!* 1-877-823-9235

Notes:

December

Blood Sugar	Sunday 12				Monday 13				Tuesday 14			
	M	N	E	B	M	N	E	B	M	N	E	B
≥ 200												
190												
180												
170												
160												
150												
140												
130												
120												
110												
100												
90												
80												
70												
≤60												

M = Morning, N = Noon, E = Evening, B = Bedtime.

December

Wednesday 15				Thursday 16				Friday 17				Saturday 18			
M	N	E	B	M	N	E	B	M	N	E	B	M	N	E	B

M = Morning, N = Noon, E = Evening, B = Bedtime.

Its time to order your new *DIABETIC DIARY 2005!* 1-877-823-9235

Notes:

December

Blood Sugar	Sunday 19				Monday 20				Tuesday 21			
	M	N	E	B	M	N	E	B	M	N	E	B
≥ 200												
190												
180												
170												
160												
150												
140												
130												
120												
110												
100												
90												
80												
70												
≤60												

M = Morning, N = Noon, E = Evening, B = Bedtime.

December

Wednesday 22				Thursday 23				Friday 24				Saturday 25			
M	N	E	B	M	N	E	B	M	N	E	B	M	N	E	B

M = Morning, N = Noon, E = Evening, B = Bedtime.

Its time to order your new *DIABETIC DIARY 2005!* 1-877-823-9235

Notes:

December

Blood Sugar	Sunday 26				Monday 27				Tuesday 28			
	M	N	E	B	M	N	E	B	M	N	E	B
≥ 200												
190												
180												
170												
160												
150												
140												
130												
120												
110												
100												
90												
80												
70												
≤60												

M = Morning, N = Noon, E = Evening, B = Bedtime.

December

Wednesday 29				Thursday 30				Friday 31				Saturday			
M	N	E	B	M	N	E	B	M	N	E	B	M	N	E	B

M = Morning, N = Noon, E = Evening, B = Bedtime.

Its time to order your new *DIABETIC DIARY 2005!* 1-877-823-9235

Notes:

Weights

▶ Checks for risk of worsening diabetes.

▶ Recording your weights monthly should be adequate.

▶ Weight management is important, especially in Type 2 diabetes. Obese Type 2 diabetics can significantly improve their blood sugar control and sometimes cure their diabetes with weight reduction. Conversely, weight gain can contribute to uncontrolled diabetes and subsequent complications.

▶ Calculate your body mass index (BMI) from the following formula:
BMI = weight _____ Kg ÷ (height _____ meters)^2 = _____

Normal is BMI ≤ 25.
Overweight is BMI between 25 and 30.
Obese is BMI ≥ 30.

▶ Conversion from English units is easy.
Weight _____ lb. ÷ 2.2 = _____ Kg.
Height _____ in. x 2.54 ÷ 100 = _____ meters.
Height^2 = _____ meters x _____ meters = _____ meters^2

Weights

	January	February	March	April
Pounds				
Kilograms				
BMI				

	May	June	July	August
Pounds				
Kilograms				
BMI				

	September	October	November	December
Pounds				
Kilograms				
BMI				

Blood Pressure

▸ Checks risk for heart disease, stroke and kidney disease.

▸ Record your blood pressures as measured by a health care professional monthly should be adequate. Your physician may monitor your blood pressure more frequently until it is under control. You may use an average if your health care provider measures several readings during one visit.

▸ Current recommendations:
   Systolic Blood Pressure ≤ 130 (top number).
   Diastolic Blood Pressure ≤ 80 (bottom number).

Blood Pressure

	January	February	March	April
Systolic mm Hg				
Diastolic mm Hg				

	May	June	July	August
Systolic mm Hg				
Diastolic mm Hg				

	September	October	November	December
Systolic mm Hg				
Diastolic mm Hg				

Hemoglobin A1C
(Glycosylated Hemoglobin)

▸ Measures average blood sugar control over the preceding 2 or 3 months.

▸ Record values in the corresponding month in which they were tested.

▸ Measurement is recommended twice yearly if sugar control is stable and quarterly if treatment goals aren't met or if therapy is changed.

▸ **As a general rule, therapeutic blood sugar control is indicated by a result of ≤ 7%. Change in therapy is indicated at values ≥ 8%.**

▸ Note: There is a lack of standardization between assays, so your doctor may make recommendations idiosyncratic to the assay used.

Hemoglobin A1C
(Glycosylated Hemoglobin)

January	%	July	%
February	%	August	%
March	%	September	%
April	%	October	%
May	%	November	%
Jun	%	December	%

Lipids

▶ Checks risk for heart disease and stroke.

▶ Record values in the corresponding month in which they were tested.

▶ Generally, adult diabetic patients should have their lipids checked yearly. Lipids that should be measured include LDL-cholesterol (bad cholesterol), HDL-cholesterol (good cholesterol) and triglycerides. Children > 2 year of age may be screened.

▶ If the resultant values fall into the low risk category (LDL-C < 100 mg/dL, HDL-C > 45 mg/dL for men and > 55 mg/dL for women, triglycerides <200) screening can be performed every 2 years.

▶ Testing may be indicated more often when being pharmacologically treated for high risk lipid levels, especially in the initiation stages.

▶ Therapeutic goals include
LDL-cholesterol < 100 mg/dL
HDL-cholesterol > 45 mg/dL for men and >55 mg/dL for women
Triglycerides < 200 mg/dL

▶ If treated pharmacologically other tests may be indicated, most commonly the transaminases ALT (alanine aminotransferase) and AST (aspartame aminotransferase) to monitor liver function and CK (creatine kinase) to monitor skeletal muscle biochemistry. Space is included for these test results.

Lipids

	January	February	March	April
LDL-C mg/dL				
HDL-C mg/dL				
Trig mg/dL				
ALT IU/dL				
AST IU/dL				
CK IU/dL				

	May	June	July	August
LDL-C mg/dL				
HDL-C mg/dL				
Trig mg/dL				
ALT IU/dL				
AST IU/dL				
CK IU/dL				

	September	October	November	December
LDL-C mg/dL				
HDL-C mg/dL				
Trig mg/dL				
ALT IU/dL				
AST IU/dL				
CK IU/dL				

Urinary Microalbumin

_____Check here if your doctor has diagnosed you with gross proteinuria and skip this section

▸ Checks kidney (renal function)

▸ Record values in the corresponding month in which they were tested.

▸ Urinalysis should be performed yearly. If no protein is detected then a follow up test should be performed looking for small amounts of albumin, called microalbumin. The test can be performed in any of three ways.
  1. Random first morning urine sample is the most common and convenient method used. If a first morning specimen is not possible, urine samples should be obtained at the same time of day for meaningful comparisons. The creatinine in the urine is also measured and the result is reported as a ratio
  Normal value is < 30 μg/mg.
  2. Twenty four hour collection. Urine is collected for 24 hours and analyzed for the total albumin.
  Normal value is <30 mg/24 hr.
  3. Timed collection over 4 or 8 hours.
  Normal value is <20 μg/min.

▸ Because of normal variability, 2 of 3 specimens over a 3 to 6 month period should be abnormal before this test is considered positive. Exercise, infection, fever, congestive heart failure, severe hyperglycemia and severe hypertension can cause false positives.

Urinary Microalbumin

	January	February	March	April
μg / mg				
mg / 24 hr.				
μg / min				

	May	June	July	August
μg / mg				
mg / 24 hr.				
μg / min				

	September	October	November	December
μg / mg				
mg / 24 hr.				
μg / min				

Kidney (renal) Function

▸ Record values in the corresponding month in which they were tested.

▸ There are no specific recommendations for testing intervals, but your physician should be checking these values, especially if you are on certain medications such as metformin (Glucophage) and ACE inhibitors.

▸ Another measurement of kidney function is blood urea nitrogen (BUN) and creatinine (CRT). Especially if you are taking a blood pressure medication called ACE inhibitors (angiotensin converting enzyme inhibitors) you should have your BUN, CRT and K (potassium) checked 2-3 weeks after initiation of the medication and 2-3 weeks after any dose change, then periodically.

Kidney (renal) Function

	January	February	March	April
BUN mg/dL				
CRT mg/dL				
K meq/dL				

	May	June	July	August
BUN mg/dL				
CRT mg/dL				
K meq/dL				

	September	October	November	December
BUN mg/dL				
CRT mg/dL				
K meq/dL				

Examinations

▶ Record your physicians names in the space provided.

▶ Check the month(s) corresponding to examination dates.

▶ **General diabetic examinations:**
  1. **Twice yearly** if your diabetes is controlled.
  2. **Quarterly** if not meeting theraputic goals. More often if prescribed.

▶ **Diabetic foot examinations:**
  1. **Your feet should be examined at every doctor visit!** It is best just to get into the habit of taking your shoes and socks off every time you see your doctor!
  2. **A yearly examination** by a foot specialist such as a *podiatrist, orthopedic surgeon or vascular surgeon* is recommended by some.

▶ **Diabetic eye examinations:**
  1. **Yearly** by an *ophthalmologist*; more often if prescribed. Diabetes is still the most common cause of blindness world wide.

GENERAL DIABETIC Examinations

January		July	
February		August	
March		September	
April		October	
May		November	
Jun		December	

Diabetic Specialist Contact Information_____

DIABETIC Foot Examinations

January		July	
February		August	
March		September	
April		October	
May		November	
Jun		December	

Diabetic Foot Specialist Contact Information_____

DIABETIC Eye Examinations

January	
February	
March	
April	
May	
Jun	

July	
August	
September	
October	
November	
December	

Ophthalmologist Contact Information_____

About the Author

L. D. Sutton, M.D., Ph.D.

Dr. Sutton is a physician-scientist with 58 scientific publications and presentations to his credit. He received his Medical Degree from the University of Iowa College of Medicine and his Doctoral of Philosophy degree from the University of Iowa College of Liberal Arts' Department of Chemistry. He completed specialty training in Clinical Pathology at the University of Iowa Hospitals and Clinics and in Family Practice at Broadlawns Medical Center in Des Moines, Iowa. His practice experience includes faculty positions in pathology at both the University of Arkansas for Medical Sciences and the University of Iowa Hospitals and Clinics, Director of Clinical Microbiology at the McClellan Memorial Veteran's Administration Hospital in Little Rock, Arkansas and a successful private practice in Family and Emergency Medicine. After serving as Senior Research Scientist for Bio-Research Products, Inc., he co-founded Joel Health Industries, Inc. where he currently works as President.

References

1. American Diabetic Association. www.diabetes.org. September 2003 review of Position statements, Consensus statements and Technical reviews.

2. American Diabetic Association. www.diabetes.org. August 2002 review of Position statements, Consensus statements and Technical reviews.

3. American Diabetic Association. www.diabetes.org. August 2001 review of Position statements, Consensus statements and Technical reviews.

4. ABCNEWS.com. Fending off the Flu, New Pill Works Like Vaccine, 20 November 2000.

5. American Family Physician. Alternative Therapies: Part I. Depression, Diabetes, Obesity. 1 September 2000.

6. American Family Physician. Diagnosis and Classification of Diabetes Mellitus New Criteria. 15 October 1998

7. American Family Physician. New Oral Therapies for Type 2 Diabetes. 1 November 1997.

8. American Family Physician. New Treatments for Diabetes. 15 May 1999.

9. American Family Physician. Oral Pharmacological of Type 2 Diabetes. 1 December 1999.

10. American Family Physician. Use of ACE Inhibitors in Patients with Type 2 Diabetes. 1 May 2000.

0-595-29875-3

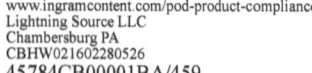